CANCER CARE FOR ADULTS

Nurturing Wellness: Holistic Strategies for Thriving Beyond Cancer

Daniel J. Contreras

Table of Contents

Part 1: Understanding Adult Cancer Care

Equipping yourself with knowledge is a powerful first step on your adult cancer care journey. This section dives into the essential aspects, guiding you through the initial phases and treatment decisions.

Here's a glimpse of what you'll learn:

- **Navigating a Diagnosis:** We'll explore what to expect after receiving a cancer diagnosis, including common tests, consultations, and strategies for coping with the emotional impact.

- **Your Care Team:** You'll discover the diverse specialists involved in adult cancer care, understand the importance of a multidisciplinary approach, and learn how to build trust and effective communication with your healthcare providers.

- **Treatment Options:** We'll delve into the common cancer treatment modalities like surgery, chemotherapy, and radiation therapy. You'll gain insights into factors influencing treatment decisions and explore the concept of setting treatment goals, whether curative, focused on symptom management, or palliative care.

This section empowers you with foundational knowledge as you embark on your adult cancer care journey.

Chapter 1: Introduction: The Landscape of Adult Cancer Care

A cancer diagnosis can be a life-altering event, but you are not alone. This chapter equips you with knowledge about the initial phase of adult cancer care, specifically what to expect after receiving a diagnosis.

1.1 Facing a Diagnosis: What to Expect

Receiving a cancer diagnosis may be terrifying and debilitating. . This section serves as a roadmap to navigate the initial stages:

- **Understanding Different Types of Cancer Diagnoses:** There are over 200 different types of cancer, each with its own characteristics and treatment approaches.

This section will provide a general overview of how cancers are categorized and diagnosed, helping you gain basic understanding of your specific diagnosis.

- **Initial Tests, Procedures, and Consultations:** Following a diagnosis, there will likely be a series of tests and consultations to confirm the diagnosis and determine the stage of the cancer. This might include blood tests, imaging scans (X-ray, CT scan, MRI), and biopsies. You'll also meet with various specialists who will discuss your condition and treatment options.

- **Emotional Impact of a Cancer Diagnosis and Coping Strategies:** A cancer diagnosis can trigger a range of emotions, including fear, anxiety, anger, and sadness.

It's important to acknowledge these emotions and develop healthy coping mechanisms. We'll explore strategies for managing difficult emotions and finding support systems.

Remember, knowledge is empowering. By understanding what to expect in the initial stages, you can approach your cancer care journey with a sense of control and focus on getting the best possible treatment.

1.2 Types of Adult Cancer Care Teams

Cancer care is a complex process, and no single doctor can manage it alone. This section highlights the importance of a multidisciplinary team approach and introduces the various specialists you might encounter in adult cancer care:

- **Oncologists:** These are doctors who specialize in diagnosing and treating cancer. There are different types of oncologists, each with a specific area of expertise.

    - **Medical Oncologists:** They typically oversee your overall care, prescribe medications like chemotherapy and targeted therapies, and manage side effects.

- **Surgical Oncologists:** They specialize in performing surgery to remove cancerous tumors.

  - **Radiation Oncologists:** These doctors use radiation therapy to target and destroy cancer cells.

- **Other Specialists:** Depending on your specific cancer type or needs, you might interact with additional specialists like:

  - **Pathologists:** These doctors examine tissue samples under a microscope to diagnose cancer and determine its characteristics.

  - **Radiologists:** They use imaging techniques like X-rays, CT scans, and MRIs to diagnose cancer and monitor treatment progress.

- **Registered Nurses:** They provide essential patient care, administer medications, and offer emotional support throughout your treatment journey.

  - **Nurse Practitioners:** These advanced practice nurses can perform many tasks typically done by a doctor, including prescribing medications and managing treatment plans.

- **The Power of a Multidisciplinary Team:** A multidisciplinary team approach ensures all aspects of your care are coordinated and addressed. Each specialist brings their unique expertise to the table, working together to create a personalized treatment plan tailored to your specific needs.

- **Building Trust and Communication:**
  Establishing open communication and trust with
  your healthcare providers is crucial. Don't
  hesitate to ask questions, voice your concerns,
  and express your preferences. The team is there
  to support you and guide you through every step
  of the way.

By understanding the composition of your adult cancer
care team and the importance of a collaborative
approach, you can feel empowered to actively participate
in your treatment decisions.

1.3 Treatment Options and Considerations

Cancer treatment has evolved significantly, offering a diverse range of options. This section explores the most common modalities and the factors influencing your treatment plan:

- **Understanding Treatment Modalities:**
  - **Surgery:** This involves physically removing cancerous tissue. There are various surgical techniques, and the type used depends on the location and stage of your cancer.
  - **Chemotherapy:** These are powerful drugs that target and kill rapidly dividing cells, including cancer cells.

Chemotherapy can be administered
intravenously, orally, or topically,
depending on the specific medication.

- **Radiation Therapy:** This uses
  high-energy rays to destroy cancer cells
  or shrink tumors. Radiation can be
  delivered externally through a machine or
  internally by placing radioactive material
  near the tumor site.

- **Factors Influencing Treatment Decisions:**
  - **Stage of Cancer:** The stage refers to the
    extent of cancer spread, impacting
    treatment choices. Early-stage cancers
    might be treated with surgery alone, while
    advanced stages may involve a
    combination of modalities.

- **Type of Cancer:** Different types of cancer respond better to specific treatments. Your doctor will consider the unique characteristics of your cancer when formulating a plan.
  - **Overall Health:** Your overall health and ability to tolerate treatment side effects will influence treatment recommendations.
- **Setting Treatment Goals:**
  - **Curative Treatment:** This aims to completely eliminate cancer cells and achieve a cure.
  - **Symptom Management:** Treatment might focus on controlling symptoms like pain or improving quality of life, even if the cancer can't be cured.

- **Palliative Care:** This provides comfort and symptom relief for advanced stages of cancer and focuses on improving the patient's quality of life.

Important Considerations:

- No single approach fits everyone. The best treatment plan is personalized based on your specific circumstances.
- Actively participate in discussions with your healthcare provider. Ask questions and understand the rationale behind each treatment option.

- There may be benefits and risks associated with each treatment modality. Weighing these factors and potential side effects is crucial for making informed decisions.

By understanding the different treatment options and the considerations involved, you can actively participate in shaping your personalized cancer care plan.

Chapter 2: Traditional Cancer Treatments

2.1 Surgery: A Closer Look

Surgery is a cornerstone of cancer treatment, often used to remove cancerous tissue and potentially cure the disease. This section delves deeper into the different types of surgeries used in adult cancer care:

- **Types of Cancer Surgery:**
    - **Curative Surgery:** This aims to completely remove all cancerous tissue, with the intent of achieving a cure.
    - **Debulking Surgery:** This removes as much of the tumor as possible, even if complete removal isn't feasible.

It can be used to alleviate symptoms, improve the effectiveness of other treatments like radiation therapy, or prepare for reconstructive surgery.

- **Reconstructive Surgery:** This surgery aims to restore function and appearance after cancer surgery, improving a patient's quality of life.

- **Preparing for Surgery:**
  - **Preoperative Consultations:** Before surgery, you'll meet with your surgeon and other specialists to discuss the procedure, potential risks and benefits, and anesthesia options.
  - **Pre-operative Tests:** You may undergo various tests like blood tests, imaging scans, and biopsies to assess your overall health and ensure you're fit for surgery.

- **The Surgical Process:**

  - **Types of Anesthesia:** Depending on the complexity of the surgery, you might receive general anesthesia (completely unconscious) or regional anesthesia (numbs a specific area of the body).

  - **Minimally Invasive Surgery:** Whenever possible, surgeons utilize minimally invasive techniques to minimize scarring and expedite recovery. This might involve laparoscopic or robotic-assisted surgery.

  - **Open Surgery:** In some cases, depending on the tumor location and size, traditional open surgery might be necessary.

- **Recovery and Side Effects:**

  - **Post-operative Care:** Following surgery, you'll receive pain management medications and instructions for wound care. The length of your hospital stay will depend on the type of surgery and your recovery progress.

  - **Potential Side Effects:** Surgery can cause side effects like pain, infection, bleeding, and fatigue. Your doctor will provide medications and strategies to manage these side effects.

- **Physical Therapy:** Depending on the surgery, you might require physical therapy to regain strength and mobility.

By understanding the different types of cancer surgery, the preoperative process, and potential side effects, you can approach surgery feeling more informed and prepared.

2.2 Demystifying Chemotherapy

Chemotherapy is a powerful weapon in the fight against cancer. This section sheds light on how it works, different types of chemotherapy drugs, and what to expect during treatment.

- **Understanding Chemotherapy:**
  Chemotherapy drugs target and destroy rapidly dividing cells, including cancer cells. Since cancer cells grow and multiply quickly, they are more susceptible to the effects of these drugs compared to healthy cells. However, chemotherapy can also affect healthy cells that divide rapidly, leading to side effects.

- **Types of Chemotherapy Drugs:**
  There are many different chemotherapy drugs, each with its own mechanism of action and side effect profile. Common types include:

- Alkylating agents: These damage the DNA of cancer cells, preventing them from dividing.

- Antimetabolites: These interfere with the production of new DNA in cancer cells.

- Vinca alkaloids: These disrupt cell division by interfering with the formation of the mitotic spindle (a structure that helps cells divide).

- Taxanes: These promote the formation of abnormal microtubules (structures that help cells divide), ultimately leading to cell death.

- Platinum-based drugs: These damage the DNA of cancer cells and interfere with their repair mechanisms.

- **Administration and Treatment Schedules:**
  Chemotherapy can be administered through
  various routes, including:
  - Intravenously (IV): This is the most
    common method, where the drugs are
    delivered directly into a vein.
  - Orally: Some chemotherapy drugs come
    in pill form that can be taken at home.
  - Topically: Certain creams or lotions
    containing chemotherapy drugs may be
    used for specific types of cancer.
- Chemotherapy is often given in cycles, with a
  period of rest in between to allow your body to
  recover from the effects of the drugs. The
  specific treatment schedule will depend on the
  type and stage of your cancer, as well as the
  specific drugs used.

- **Common Side Effects of Chemotherapy:**
  While chemotherapy is effective in killing cancer cells, it can also cause side effects. Some common side effects include:
  - Nausea and vomiting
  - Fatigue
  - Hair loss
  - Loss of appetite
  - Mouth sores
  - Increased risk of infection
  - Easy bruising and bleeding
- It's critical to keep in mind that every person reacts to side effects differently.. Your doctor will develop strategies to manage these side effects and improve your comfort throughout treatment.

By understanding how chemotherapy works, the different types of drugs, and potential side effects, you can approach this treatment with a sense of awareness and work with your healthcare team to manage any challenges that may arise.

2.3 Radiation Therapy: Understanding Its Role

Radiation therapy is another powerful tool used to fight cancer. This section dives into the science behind radiation therapy, the different types used in adult cancer care, and what to expect during treatment.

- **The Science of Radiation Therapy:**

Radiation therapy uses high-energy rays, such as X-rays, gamma rays, or particle beams, to target and destroy cancer cells. These rays damage the DNA of cancer cells, preventing them from dividing and growing. Unlike chemotherapy, which affects rapidly dividing cells throughout the body, radiation therapy can be targeted to a specific area, minimizing damage to healthy tissues.

- **Types of Radiation Therapy:**

There are two main types of radiation therapy used in adult cancer care:

External Beam Radiation Therapy: This is the most common type. A machine outside the body directs high-energy rays towards the cancerous tumor. Modern techniques allow for precise targeting of the radiation beam, minimizing exposure to healthy tissues.

Internal Radiation Therapy (Brachytherapy): This involves placing radioactive material sealed in a capsule or implant directly inside the body, near the tumor site. The radioactive material emits radiation that destroys nearby cancer cells.

- **Treatment Planning and Delivery:**

The radiation therapy team, including radiation oncologists, dosimetrists, and therapists, will work together to create a personalized treatment plan. This plan considers factors like the type and size of your cancer, its location, and your overall health. Imaging scans like CT scans are used to map the treatment area and create a three-dimensional picture of the tumor.

Based on this information, the team determines the precise dose of radiation needed and the treatment schedule.

The actual delivery of radiation therapy is painless. You will be positioned on a treatment table, and the radiation machine will be directed at the targeted area. Treatments typically take a few minutes and are usually given on an outpatient basis, five days a week for several weeks.

- **Potential Side Effects:**

Radiation therapy can cause side effects, depending on the area being treated. Common side effects might include:

* Skin irritation or redness in the treated area
* Fatigue
* Hair loss in the treated area
* Nausea and vomiting
* Mouth sores (if radiation is directed to the head and neck)

These side effects are usually temporary and manageable with medication and supportive care. Your doctor will discuss potential side effects in detail and provide strategies to minimize discomfort throughout treatment.

By understanding how radiation therapy works, the different types used, and potential side effects, you can approach this treatment with a sense of awareness and actively participate in discussions about your personalized treatment plan.

2.4 Clinical Trials: Exploring New Possibilities

While traditional treatments like surgery, chemotherapy, and radiation therapy form the backbone of cancer care, research continues to explore new and innovative approaches. Clinical trials play a vital role in this advancement, offering patients the opportunity to participate in testing promising new treatments.

- **The Role of Clinical Trials:**

Clinical trials are research studies designed to evaluate the safety and effectiveness of new drugs, therapies, or treatment combinations for cancer. They are conducted in a structured manner, following strict ethical guidelines to protect patient safety.

Clinical trials play a crucial role in:

* Developing new and potentially more effective cancer treatments.
* Improving existing treatment methods by refining protocols and reducing side effects.
* Gaining insights into the biology of cancer and how it responds to different therapies.

- **Understanding Different Phases of Clinical Trials:**

Clinical trials progress through different phases to ensure the safety and efficacy of new treatments:

Phase I Trials: These involve a small group of patients to assess the safety and determine the appropriate dosage of a new treatment.

Phase II Trials: These studies involve a larger group of patients to evaluate the effectiveness of the treatment for a specific type of cancer.

Phase III Trials: These are larger-scale studies that compare the new treatment with a standard treatment to determine its effectiveness and identify any potential benefits or drawbacks.

Phase IV Trials: These studies are conducted after a treatment has been approved by regulatory agencies to monitor its long-term effects and gather additional data.

- **Eligibility Criteria:**

Not everyone can participate in a clinical trial. Each trial has specific eligibility criteria based on factors like the type and stage of cancer, age, overall health, and prior treatments received. Your doctor will discuss whether a clinical trial might be a good option for you based on your individual circumstances.

- **Weighing the Benefits and Risks:**

Clinical trials offer the potential to access cutting-edge treatments before they are widely available. However, it's important to weigh the benefits and risks carefully before deciding to participate. Some potential benefits include access to new therapies, potential for improved outcomes, and contributing to scientific advancement.

On the other hand, there are also potential risks, such as side effects that may not be fully known, the possibility that the new treatment may not be effective, and the uncertainty of being assigned to the control group receiving standard treatment.

- **Making an Informed Decision:**

If you're considering participating in a clinical trial, discuss it thoroughly with your doctor. Ask questions about the specific trial, its goals, potential benefits and risks, and what to expect throughout the study. Ultimately, the decision to participate in a clinical trial is a personal one, and you should feel comfortable and well-informed before making your choice.

By understanding the role of clinical trials, the different phases involved, and the factors to consider, you can make an informed decision about whether participating in a trial might be right for you on your adult cancer care journey.

Chapter 3: Beyond Traditional Treatments: A Holistic Approach

Traditional cancer treatments like surgery, chemotherapy, and radiation therapy are powerful tools, but they are not the only weapons in your arsenal. This chapter delves into the importance of a holistic approach to cancer care, highlighting the role of nutrition in supporting your well-being throughout treatment.

3.1 The Importance of Nutrition During Cancer Care

Proper nutrition plays a critical role in your overall health and well-being, and this becomes even more crucial during cancer care. Here's why:

- **Maintaining Strength and Energy:** Cancer treatments can be physically demanding, and proper nutrition provides the essential building blocks your body needs to maintain strength and energy levels to cope with treatment and recovery.

- **Supporting Immune Function:** A healthy diet rich in vitamins, minerals, and antioxidants can strengthen your immune system, helping your body fight off infections and recover more effectively.

- **Managing Side Effects:** Many cancer treatments can cause side effects like nausea, vomiting, and loss of appetite. Eating a balanced and nutritious diet can help manage these side effects and improve your overall quality of life.

- **Promoting Treatment Effectiveness:** Proper nutrition can help your body better tolerate treatments and potentially improve their effectiveness.

Building a Healthy Eating Plan During Cancer Care

While there's no single "cancer-fighting" diet, focusing on a balanced and nutritious approach is key. Here are some tips for building a healthy eating plan during cancer care:

- **Focus on Whole Foods:** Choose whole, unprocessed foods like fruits, vegetables, whole grains, lean protein sources, and healthy fats.
- **Variety is Key:** Include a wide variety of colorful fruits and vegetables in your diet to get a full spectrum of essential vitamins, minerals, and antioxidants.

- **Stay Hydrated:** Drinking plenty of water throughout the day is crucial for overall health and can help manage side effects like fatigue and constipation.

- **Small Frequent Meals:** Eating smaller, more frequent meals may be easier to tolerate than large meals, especially if you're experiencing nausea or loss of appetite.

Addressing Specific Challenges

Cancer treatments can present unique dietary challenges. Here's how to address some common concerns:

- **Managing Nausea and Vomiting:** Certain foods like ginger, bland foods like crackers, and cold or chilled foods can help ease nausea. Talk to your doctor or a registered dietitian about anti-nausea medication if needed.

- **Coping with Loss of Appetite:** Focus on high-calorie, nutrient-dense foods like smoothies or protein shakes. Explore different flavors and textures to find appealing options.

- **Managing Mouth Sores:** Soft, bland foods like mashed potatoes, yogurt, or applesauce may be easier to tolerate with mouth sores.

Working with a Registered Dietitian

A registered dietitian can be a valuable asset on your cancer care journey. They can help you create a personalized nutrition plan that considers your specific needs, preferences, and treatment side effects. They can also provide guidance on managing dietary challenges and ensure you're getting all the essential nutrients your body needs to support healing and recovery.

By prioritizing good nutrition and working with a healthcare professional, you can empower yourself to take an active role in your well-being throughout cancer care. The following sections of this chapter will explore other aspects of a holistic approach, such as exercise, mind-body practices, and complementary therapies.

3.2 Exercise and Movement for Overall Well Being

A cancer patient's physical and mental health may suffer throughout therapy.However, incorporating regular exercise and movement into your routine can be a powerful tool to combat fatigue, improve mood, and enhance your overall well-being during and after cancer care.

Benefits of Exercise During Cancer Care:

- **Increased Physical Strength and Endurance:** Regular exercise helps maintain muscle mass and bone density, which can be depleted by some treatments. Improved strength and endurance can make it easier to manage daily activities and cope with treatment side effects like fatigue.

- **Enhanced Emotional Well-being:** Exercise releases endorphins, natural mood elevators that can combat feelings of depression and anxiety often associated with cancer.Exercise can also lower stress levels and enhance the quality of sleep.

- **Boosted Immune Function:** Regular exercise can strengthen your immune system, helping your body fight off infections and recover more effectively from treatment.

- **Reduced Risk of Long-Term Complications:** Maintaining a physically active lifestyle can help manage your weight and potentially reduce the risk of developing certain long-term complications associated with cancer and its treatment.

Safe and Effective Exercise Options:

The type and intensity of exercise you choose will depend on your overall health, fitness level, and any limitations you may have due to treatment. Here are some safe and effective options to consider:

- **Walking:** This is a low-impact, accessible activity that most people can participate in, regardless of fitness level As you become stronger, start out slowly and then increase the duration and intensity.

- **Swimming:** This is a gentle and low-impact exercise that's easy on your joints yet provides a full-body workout.

- **Yoga:** Yoga combines physical postures, breathing exercises, and meditation, promoting flexibility, strength, and relaxation. Certain yoga styles are specifically designed for individuals with cancer.

- **Tai Chi:** This mind-body practice involves slow, gentle movements and focused breathing. Tai Chi can improve balance, flexibility, and overall well-being.

- **Strength Training:** Building muscle strength can significantly improve your energy levels, functional ability, and overall sense of well-beingAs you gain strength, progressively increase the intensity of your bodyweight or light weight exercises.

Getting Started and Overcoming Challenges:

- **Talk to Your Doctor:** Before starting any new exercise program, discuss it with your doctor to ensure it's safe for you, considering your specific condition and any treatment limitations.

- **Start Slowly and Listen to Your Body:** Begin with short, manageable exercise sessions and gradually increase the duration and intensity as you feel stronger.Observe your body and take days off as necessary.

- **Find Activities You Enjoy:** The key to consistency is finding exercise activities you genuinely enjoy. Investigate many choices until you find the one that suits you the most.

- **Incorporate Movement Throughout Your Day:** Even small bursts of activity can make a difference.

Take the stairs instead of the elevator, go for short walks throughout the day, or do some gentle stretches at your desk.

By incorporating regular exercise and movement into your routine, you can become an active participant in your well-being journey during cancer care. The following section will explore the role of mind-body practices in managing stress and promoting emotional well-being.

3.3 Mind-Body Practices for Stress Management

Cancer diagnosis and treatment can be a stressful and emotionally challenging experience. This section explores mind-body practices, a powerful approach to managing stress, promoting relaxation, and fostering emotional well-being during cancer care.

The Mind-Body Connection:

Our minds and bodies are intricately linked. Stress can manifest physically, leading to symptoms like fatigue, headaches, and muscle tension. Conversely, techniques that promote relaxation and emotional well-being can have positive physical effects. Mind-body practices help bridge this gap.

Benefits of Mind-Body Practices:

- **Reduced Stress and Anxiety:** Practices like meditation and mindfulness can help calm the mind, quiet racing thoughts, and reduce feelings of overwhelm often associated with cancer.

- **Improved Sleep Quality:** Stress can disrupt sleep patterns. Mind-body practices can promote relaxation and improve your ability to fall asleep and stay asleep.

- **Enhanced Emotional Well-being:** These techniques can help you develop coping mechanisms for managing difficult emotions like fear, anger, and sadness that may arise during cancer care.

- **Increased Feelings of Control and Empowerment:** Mind-body practices can empower you to take charge of your emotional well-being and feel more in control during a challenging time.

Examples of Mind-Body Practices:

- **Meditation:** Meditation involves focusing your attention on the present moment and training your mind to become more aware of your thoughts and feelings without judgment. There are various meditation techniques, including mindfulness meditation and guided imagery.

- **Relaxation Techniques:** Deep breathing exercises, progressive muscle relaxation, and visualization techniques can help reduce stress and promote feelings of calm.

- **Yoga and Tai Chi:** These mind-body practices combine physical postures, breathing exercises, and meditation, promoting relaxation, stress reduction, and improved flexibility.

- **Mindfulness-Based Stress Reduction (MBSR):** This evidence-based program combines meditation, mindful movement, and group discussion to help manage stress and improve emotional well-being.

Getting Started with Mind-Body Practices:

There are many resources available to help you get started with mind-body practices:

- **Online Resources:** Numerous websites and apps offer guided meditations, relaxation techniques, and mindfulness exercises.

- **Support Groups:** Connecting with others who understand the challenges of cancer can be a source of support and encouragement. Some support groups may incorporate mind-body practices into their meetings.

- **Classes and Workshops:** Many hospitals, community centers, and yoga studios offer classes specifically designed for individuals with cancer.

By incorporating mind-body practices into your routine, you can equip yourself with powerful tools to manage stress, improve your emotional well-being, and navigate the challenges of cancer care with greater resilience. The following section will explore complementary and integrative therapies that may complement your traditional treatment plan.

3.4 Complementary and Integrative Therapies: Exploring Options

Alongside traditional cancer treatments and the holistic practices explored earlier, complementary and integrative therapies (CAM) offer additional avenues to support your well-being during cancer care. This section delves into what CAM therapies are and how they might complement your treatment plan.

Understanding CAM Therapies:

Complementary and integrative therapies encompass a wide range of approaches that fall outside the realm of conventional medicine. These therapies aim to:

- Improve symptoms and side effects associated with cancer treatment.
- Enhance overall well-being and quality of life.
- Support the body's natural healing mechanisms.

It's important to note that CAM therapies are not meant to replace traditional cancer treatments. The best approach often involves integrating complementary therapies alongside your standard medical care plan.

Examples of CAM Therapies:

There are numerous CAM therapies, each with its own philosophy and approach. Here are a few examples:

- **Acupuncture:** This traditional Chinese medicine technique involves inserting thin needles into specific points on the body to stimulate energy flow and potentially alleviate pain, manage nausea, and improve sleep.

- **Massage Therapy:** Massage can help reduce muscle tension, improve relaxation, and promote feelings of well-being. Specific massage techniques may be tailored to address treatment-related pain or fatigue.

- **Mindfulness-Based Stress Reduction (MBSR):** Previously discussed in section 3.3, MBSR combines meditation, mindful movement, and group discussion to manage stress and improve emotional well-being.

- **Herbal Medicine:** Certain herbs and botanical supplements may offer symptom relief, but it's crucial to consult with your doctor before using any herbal products to ensure they are safe and don't interact with your cancer treatment.

Exploring CAM Therapies with Caution:

While CAM therapies can be beneficial, it's important to approach them with caution:

- **Research the Therapy:** Gather information about the specific CAM therapy you're considering, including its potential benefits, risks, and scientific evidence supporting its use.
- **Consult Your Doctor:** Always discuss any CAM therapy with your doctor before starting it. They can help you understand how it might interact with your traditional treatment plan and ensure its safety for you.

- **Beware of Unrealistic Claims:** Avoid therapies that promise miraculous cures or seem too good to be true. Focus on therapies that aim to support your well-being and manage symptoms alongside conventional treatment.

Finding a Qualified Practitioner:

If you decide to explore CAM therapies, find a qualified and experienced practitioner. Look for practitioners certified by reputable organizations specific to the type of therapy you're interested in.

By exploring complementary and integrative therapies with a cautious and informed approach, you can potentially enhance your well-being and empower yourself to take an active role in managing your cancer care journey.

Part 2: Thriving Beyond Cancer

Having navigated the initial phases of cancer care and treatment, you're now positioned to focus on thriving beyond the diagnosis. This section equips you with tools and strategies to:

- **Manage Long-Term Effects:** Explore potential long-term effects of treatments and strategies for managing them.

- **Embrace Survivorship:** Learn about the unique challenges and opportunities associated with cancer survivorship.

- **Maintain a Healthy Lifestyle:** Discover how to adopt healthy habits for long-term well-being and potentially reduce the risk of recurrence.

- **Reconnect with Life:** Explore strategies for reintegrating into your life after cancer treatment and rediscovering your sense of purpose.

- **Navigate Emotional Well-being:** Gain insights into managing emotional challenges that may arise after treatment and strategies for fostering emotional resilience.

This section empowers you to move forward with a positive outlook, focusing on living a full and meaningful life beyond cancer.

Chapter 4: Managing the Emotional Journey

Cancer can be a life-altering experience, triggering a range of emotions. This chapter delves into strategies for coping with fear, anxiety, and depression, common emotional challenges that may arise throughout your cancer journey.

4.1 Coping with Fear, Anxiety, and Depression

A cancer diagnosis can evoke a sense of fear and uncertainty about the future. It's normal to experience these emotions. However, if left unmanaged, they can significantly impact your well-being.

Here are strategies for coping with fear, anxiety, and depression:

- **Acknowledge Your Feelings:** Trying to suppress your emotions won't make them go away. Allow yourself to feel your emotions, validate them, and express them in healthy ways.It can be beneficial to speak with a therapist, support group, family member, or trusted friend.

- **Learn About Your Cancer:** Knowledge is empowering. Educate yourself about your specific type of cancer, treatment options, and potential side effects. Reliable sources like the American Cancer Society or the National Cancer Institute can provide accurate information.

- **Focus on What You Can Control:** Cancer may feel overwhelming, but you can focus on aspects you can control.

This might involve creating a healthy routine, prioritizing self-care activities, or participating actively in your treatment decisions.

- **Practice Relaxation Techniques:** Mind-body practices like meditation, deep breathing exercises, and progressive muscle relaxation can help manage stress and anxiety. These techniques can promote feelings of calm and improve your ability to cope with challenging emotions.

- **Maintain a Healthy Lifestyle:** Eating a balanced diet, getting regular exercise, and ensuring adequate sleep can significantly improve your mood and overall well-being.

When to Seek Professional Help

While it's normal to experience emotional challenges during cancer care, sometimes these feelings can become overwhelming and interfere with your daily life. Here are signs that indicate seeking professional help might be beneficial:

- Feeling overwhelmed by fear, anxiety, or sadness for extended periods.
- Difficulty sleeping or changes in appetite.
- Loss of enthusiasm for things you used to appreciate.
- Difficulty concentrating or making decisions.
- Thoughts of self-harm or suicide.

If you experience any of these signs, don't hesitate to seek professional help from a therapist or counselor.

They can provide support, teach coping mechanisms, and help you develop strategies for managing difficult emotions.

By acknowledging your feelings, adopting healthy coping strategies, and seeking professional help when needed, you can navigate the emotional challenges of cancer and emerge stronger.

The following sections of this chapter will explore additional aspects of managing the emotional journey, such as building resilience, finding meaning and purpose after cancer, and navigating relationships with loved ones.

4.2 Communication Strategies: Talking to Loved Ones

Cancer can affect not only you but also your loved ones. Open and honest communication with family and friends can be a powerful tool for fostering support and strengthening your emotional well-being throughout your cancer journey. This section equips you with strategies for talking to loved ones about your diagnosis, treatment, and emotional needs.

The Importance of Communication:

- **Reduced Stress and Anxiety:** Sharing your feelings and concerns with loved ones can provide emotional support and alleviate feelings of isolation.

- **Stronger Support System:** Open communication allows your loved ones to understand your needs and offer support in ways that are most beneficial to you.

- **Improved Decision-Making:** Having open conversations with loved ones can help you navigate treatment options and feel empowered during decision-making processes.

Initiating the Conversation:

- **Choose the Right Time and Place:** Find a quiet, private space where you can have a conversation without interruptions.

- **Start by Sharing Your Diagnosis:** Be honest and direct about your diagnosis in a way that feels comfortable for you.

- **Express Your Needs:** Let your loved ones know how they can best support you, whether it's emotional support, practical help with errands or childcare, or simply being a listening ear.

Tips for Effective Communication:

- **Use "I" Statements:** Focus on how you're feeling rather than placing blame. For instance, it works better to say, "I'm afraid of the surgery," than, "This surgery is stressing me out."

- **Be Clear and Direct:** Avoid sugar coating your feelings or using medical jargon that your loved ones might not understand.

- **Encourage Questions:** Welcome questions from your loved ones and address their concerns honestly.

- **Set Boundaries:** It's okay to set boundaries about how much information you want to share or how much company you can handle at a time.

Coping with Difficult Conversations:

- **Prepare for Different Reactions:** Everyone reacts differently to difficult news. Be patient and understanding if your loved ones have strong emotional responses.

- **Address Disagreements:** There might be times when you and your loved ones disagree about treatment options or your level of involvement in decision-making.Find common ground by being upfront with each other and communicating.

- **Seek Support for Communication Challenges:** If you're struggling to communicate effectively with loved ones, consider talking to a therapist or counselor who can provide guidance on navigating these conversations.

By prioritizing open and honest communication with your loved ones, you can build a stronger support system and navigate the emotional challenges of cancer with greater resilience. The following sections of this chapter will explore building resilience, finding meaning and purpose after cancer, and navigating intimacy and sexuality.

4.3 Finding Support Groups and Resources

Cancer can be a lonely journey, but you don't have to face it alone. Connecting with others who understand the challenges you're going through can be a source of invaluable support, encouragement, and shared experiences. This section highlights the importance of support groups and resources available to you throughout your cancer care journey.

Benefits of Support Groups:

- **Emotional Support:** Sharing your experiences with others who understand what you're going through can provide a sense of validation and belonging.

- **Reduced Isolation:** Connecting with others fighting cancer can help alleviate feelings of isolation and loneliness.

- **Practical Advice:** Support groups can be a valuable source of practical advice on coping with side effects, managing treatment, and navigating the healthcare system.

- **Hope and Inspiration:** Hearing stories of successful cancer journeys from others can provide hope and inspiration for your own path.

Types of Support Groups:

There are many different types of support groups available, catering to specific needs and preferences. Here are a few examples:

- **Cancer-Specific Support Groups:** These groups connect individuals with the same type of cancer, allowing for targeted discussions about treatment options, side effects, and emotional challenges specific to that particular cancer.

- **Treatment-Specific Support Groups:** These groups focus on supporting individuals undergoing a specific treatment, such as chemotherapy or radiation therapy.

- **Online Support Groups:** Online platforms offer virtual support groups where you can connect with others from the comfort of your home.

Finding a Support Group:

Many resources can help you find a support group that's right for you. Here are some starting points:

- **Hospitals and Cancer Treatment Centers:** Many hospitals and treatment centers offer support groups for their patients.

- **Cancer Organizations:** Organizations like the American Cancer Society and the National Cancer Institute offer information and resources for finding support groups in your area.

- **Online Resources:** Several online resources can help you locate support groups, including the National Cancer Institute's Support Group Directory and CancerCare

Additional Resources:

Beyond support groups, numerous resources are available to provide information, guidance, and emotional support throughout your cancer journey. Here are some examples:

- **Cancer Organizations:** Organizations like the American Cancer Society and the National Cancer Institute offer a wealth of information about different types of cancer, treatment options, and coping strategies.

- **Therapists and Counselors:** Mental health professionals can provide valuable support in managing emotional challenges, developing coping mechanisms, and fostering resilience.

- **Online Resources:** Many reputable websites and apps offer information about cancer, treatment options, and emotional well-being.

Remember: Don't hesitate to reach out for support. There's no shame in asking for help. By connecting with support groups and resources, you can empower yourself to navigate the challenges of cancer with greater strength and a renewed sense of hope.

Chapter 5: Life After Treatment: Regaining Strength and Redefining Normal

Treatment for cancer is often successful, but it can also leave behind long-term side effects. This chapter equips you with strategies for managing these effects and reclaiming your sense of normalcy after treatment is complete.

5.1 Managing Long-Term Side Effects

The fight against cancer doesn't end with the completion of treatment. Many people experience long-term side effects that can impact their physical and emotional well-being. Here's what you can expect:

- **Understanding Your Specific Risks:** Talk to your doctor about the potential long-term side effects associated with your specific cancer and its treatment. This awareness can help you prepare and manage these effects proactively.

- **Common Long-Term Side Effects:** These may include fatigue, pain, anxiety, depression, cognitive changes, sleep problems, and sexual dysfunction. The specific effects will vary depending on the type of cancer and treatment received.

- **Developing a Management Plan:** Work with your healthcare team to develop a plan to manage your long-term side effects. This may involve medication, physical therapy, occupational therapy, psychological counseling, or other interventions.

Here are some specific strategies for managing common long-term side effects:

- **Fatigue:** Prioritize getting enough sleep, practice relaxation techniques, and pace yourself throughout the day.

- **Pain:** Talk to your doctor about pain management strategies, which may include medication, physical therapy, or alternative therapies like acupuncture.

- **Anxiety and Depression:** Consider relaxation techniques like meditation or deep breathing exercises. Therapy can also be helpful in managing these emotional challenges.

- **Cognitive Changes:** Maintain a mentally stimulating lifestyle, play brain games, and keep yourself organized with planners or to-do lists.

- **Sleep Problems:** Develop a regular sleep schedule, create a relaxing bedtime routine, and ensure a comfortable sleep environment.

- **Sexual Dysfunction:** Open communication with your partner is key. Talk to your doctor about treatment options or rehabilitation techniques that may improve sexual function.

5.2 Building a Healthy Lifestyle for Post-Cancer Wellness

Your body may experience side effects from cancer treatment. But once treatment is complete, focusing on a healthy lifestyle becomes even more crucial. By adopting healthy habits, you can:

- Improve your overall well-being and physical fitness.

- Reduce the risk of recurrence for certain cancers.

- Manage long-term side effects and improve your quality of life.

- Increase your vitality and make you feel your best.

Here are some key pillars of a healthy lifestyle to prioritize after cancer treatment:

- **Balanced Nutrition:**

  - Focus on whole, unprocessed foods like fruits, vegetables, whole grains, lean proteins, and healthy fats.
  - Choose nutrient-dense foods that provide your body with the building blocks it needs to heal and recover.
  - Drink lots of water to stay hydrated throughout the day.

- **Regular Exercise:**

  - Aim for at least 150 minutes of moderate-intensity exercise or 75 minutes of vigorous-intensity exercise per week.

  - Consider activities you enjoy, such as walking, swimming, biking, yoga, or dancing.

  - Start slowly and gradually increase the intensity and duration of your workouts as you feel stronger.

- **Quality Sleep:**

  - Aim for 7-8 hours of quality sleep each night.

  - Establish a regular sleep schedule and practice a relaxing bedtime routine to promote better sleep.

- **Stress Management:**

  - Chronic stress can negatively impact your health.

  - Techniques like meditation, deep breathing exercises, and mindfulness practices can help manage stress and promote relaxation.

- **Weight Management:**

  - Maintaining a healthy weight can reduce the risk of certain cancers and improve overall health.

  - Focus on healthy eating and regular exercise to manage your weight effectively.

Additional Tips:

- **Limit Alcohol Consumption:** Excessive alcohol consumption can increase the risk of certain cancers and negatively impact your health.

- **Don't Smoke:** Smoking significantly increases the risk of cancer and other health problems.Giving up smoking is one of the best things you can do for your health if you smoke.

- **Sun Protection:** Protect your skin from harmful UV rays by wearing sunscreen with SPF 30 or higher daily, even on cloudy days.

- **Regular Cancer Screenings:** Continue with recommended cancer screenings as advised by your doctor.

- **Listen to Your Body:** Pay attention to your body's signals and adjust your activity level and rest periods as needed.

By making healthy choices a priority, you can empower yourself to thrive after cancer treatment and live a long and fulfilling life. The following section of this chapter will explore strategies for reintegrating back into work and social life, discovering a renewed sense of purpose, and embracing survivorship.

5.3 Creating a New Normal: Rediscovering Purpose

Cancer can be a life-altering experience, forcing you to re-evaluate your priorities and values. This section explores strategies for rediscovering your sense of purpose and creating a new normal as you move forward after treatment.

Redefining Normal:

- **Acknowledge the Changes:** Cancer and its treatment may have changed your physical and emotional capabilities. Accepting these changes is crucial for redefining your "normal" and setting realistic expectations.

- **Focus on What Matters Most:** Cancer can serve as a wake-up call to prioritize what truly matters to you in life. Reflect on your values, passions, and goals, and explore ways to integrate them into your new normal.

Finding Purpose and Meaning:

- **Explore Your Passions:** Have you always wanted to learn a new skill, volunteer for a cause you care about, or travel the world? Now might be the perfect time to pursue those passions and find activities that bring you joy and fulfillment.

- **Help Others:** Helping others can be a powerful source of purpose. Consider volunteering your time or expertise to a cause close to your heart or mentoring someone facing a similar challenge.

- **Focus on Relationships:** Nurture your relationships with loved ones who have supported you throughout your journey. Strong social connections are essential for emotional well-being and a sense of belonging.

- **Embrace Personal Growth:** Cancer can be a catalyst for personal growth. Use this experience to learn more about yourself, develop new skills, and appreciate the preciousness of life.

Creating a Fulfilling Life After Cancer:

- **Set Realistic Goals:**Divide your most ambitious objectives into more manageable chunks. Acknowledge your accomplishments along the way, and don't be scared to modify your objectives when necessary.

- **Practice Gratitude:** Focusing on the positive aspects of your life, even the small things, can cultivate a sense of gratitude and appreciation for each day.

- **Maintain a Positive Outlook:** A positive outlook can significantly impact your well-being. Focus on the possibilities that lie ahead and the opportunities to create a fulfilling life beyond cancer.

This concludes Chapter 5: Life After Treatment: Regaining Strength and Redefining Normal. The following chapters will likely delve deeper into specific aspects of survivorship, such as navigating intimacy and sexuality, managing financial challenges, and advocating for yourself in the healthcare system.

Chapter 6: Advocacy and Empowerment

Having navigated cancer treatment and begun to rebuild your life, you now possess the knowledge and experience to become an advocate for yourself and others facing similar challenges. This chapter empowers you to understand your rights as a patient and equips you with tools to navigate the healthcare system effectively.

6.1 Understanding Your Rights as a Patient

Empowered patients take an active role in their healthcare decisions. Understanding your rights as a patient is the foundation for effective advocacy:

- **Right to Information:** You have the right to clear and understandable information about your diagnosis, treatment options, potential side effects, and risks and benefits of each option. Don't hesitate to ask questions and seek clarification until you feel comfortable with the information provided.

- **Right to Informed Consent:** Before undergoing any treatment procedure, you have the right to informed consent.

This means receiving all relevant information about the procedure, its potential risks and benefits, and alternative treatment options. Only with this information can you provide your informed consent to proceed.

- **Right to Refuse Treatment:** You have the right to refuse any treatment option, even if it's recommended by your doctor. The decision ultimately rests with you, and your doctor should respect your wishes.

- **Right to Privacy:** Your medical records are confidential. You have the right to control who has access to them and to request copies for your own records.

- **Right to a Second Opinion:** You have the right to seek a second opinion from another healthcare professional before making any major treatment decisions.

6.2 Cancer Research and Staying Informed on Advancements

The field of cancer research is constantly evolving, offering renewed hope for improved treatments and potential cures. This section empowers you to stay informed about these advancements and navigate the ever-changing landscape of cancer care.

The Importance of Staying Informed:

Empowerment: Knowledge is power. Staying informed about the latest research and treatment options allows you to participate actively in your healthcare decisions and explore potential avenues for managing your cancer.

Hope and Inspiration: Learning about breakthroughs and ongoing clinical trials can provide a sense of hope and optimism for the future of cancer treatment.

Advocacy: By staying informed about research developments, you can become a more effective advocate for yourself and others facing cancer.

Finding Reliable Sources of Information:

With an abundance of information available online, it's crucial to rely on credible sources for accurate and up-to-date information about cancer research:

National Cancer Institute (NCI): The NCI website provides comprehensive information about different types of cancer, treatment options, ongoing clinical trials, and the latest research advancements.

American Cancer Society (ACS): The ACS website offers patient-friendly resources on various cancer topics, including information about clinical trials and new treatment developments.

Cancer Research Institute (CRI): The CRI website focuses on breakthroughs in cancer immunotherapy research and provides updates on promising new therapies.

ClinicalTrials.gov: This is a US government website that lists ongoing clinical trials for various diseases, including cancer.

Staying Informed While Being Mindful:

Focus on Reputable Sources: Be wary of sensationalized information or claims from unverified sources. Stick to reputable organizations and scientific journals for accurate data.

Maintain a Positive Outlook: While staying informed is important, don't overwhelm yourself with every new development. Focus on credible sources and prioritize information that directly relates to your specific situation.

Open Communication with Doctor: Discuss any research findings or clinical trials that interest you with your doctor. They can help you interpret the information and determine if it's relevant to your care plan.

The following section of this chapter will explore navigating the healthcare system, finding your voice as a patient advocate, and supporting ongoing cancer research efforts.

6.3 Building a Supportive Community: Advocacy Beyond Yourself

Cancer advocacy extends beyond understanding your rights and staying informed. This section highlights the power of building a supportive community and becoming a voice for change in the fight against cancer.

The Strength of Community:

- **Collective Action:** By joining forces with other patients, survivors, and advocates, you can amplify your voice and create a powerful movement for change.

- **Support and Networking:** Connecting with others who share similar experiences can provide emotional support, share valuable information, and foster a sense of belonging.

- **Advocacy Efforts:** Community groups can advocate for improved access to treatment, increased funding for cancer research, and better support services for patients and survivors.

Getting Involved in Advocacy:

There are numerous ways to get involved in cancer advocacy and build a supportive community:

- **Cancer Support Organizations:** Many organizations offer support groups, educational resources, and advocacy opportunities. Examples include the American Cancer Society and the National Cancer Institute

- **Patient Advocacy Groups:** These groups focus specifically on advocating for policy changes and raising awareness about specific types of cancer.

- **Online Communities:** Numerous online platforms connect patients, survivors, and caregivers, fostering a sense of community and offering opportunities to share experiences and support each other.

Finding Your Voice as an Advocate:

- **Share Your Story:** Sharing your personal experience with cancer can raise awareness and inspire others facing similar challenges. You can share your story through online platforms, support groups, or community events.

- **Contact Your Representatives:** Let your elected officials know about the issues that matter to you. Advocate for policies that improve access to quality cancer care, increase funding for research, and support patients' rights.

- **Volunteer Your Time and Skills:** Many organizations rely on volunteers to help with fundraising events, educational programs, or administrative tasks.Give off your time and expertise to change the world.

Remember: Every voice counts in the fight against cancer. By building a supportive community and getting involved in advocacy efforts, you can make a positive impact on the lives of others facing this disease, contribute to a future with better treatment options, and bring hope to those battling cancer.

The concluding section of Chapter 6 might explore additional aspects of advocacy, such as fundraising for cancer research or participating in clinical trials.

Part 3: Conclusion

Chapter 7: A Final Note: Hope and Resilience on Your Cancer Journey

Cancer is a challenging journey, filled with uncertainties and moments of fear. However, it's also a journey of immense strength, resilience, and the discovery of an inner fortitude you never knew you possessed. This concluding chapter offers a message of hope and encouragement as you navigate the path forward.

Hope is a Powerful Force:

A cancer diagnosis can feel overwhelming, but hope is a vital force that can sustain you throughout your journey. Hope fuels your determination to fight, motivates you to embrace treatment, and allows you to envision a brighter future.

- **Focus on the Positive:** Seek out stories of successful cancer survivorship, celebrate milestones along your treatment journey, and nurture a positive outlook for the future.

- **Find Inspiration:** Let the courage and resilience of others who have battled cancer inspire you. Surround yourself with positive influences who will support your emotional well-being.

Resilience: The Key to Overcoming Challenges:

Cancer can test your resilience, but it can also reveal a strength you never knew you had. Resilience is the ability to bounce back from adversity and adapt to challenging circumstances. Here's how to cultivate resilience:

- **Embrace a Support System:** Surround yourself with loving and supportive family, friends, and healthcare professionals who will champion you throughout your journey.

- **Develop Coping Mechanisms:** Learn healthy coping strategies for managing stress, anxiety, and difficult emotions. Techniques like meditation, relaxation exercises, and spending time in nature can be immensely helpful.

- **Practice Self-Compassion:** Be kind to yourself.Good days and bad days will come. Allow yourself to feel your emotions, and celebrate your victories, no matter how small.

A Life Beyond Cancer:

Cancer may have been a significant part of your journey, but it doesn't define you. As you move forward, embrace the possibilities for a fulfilling life beyond cancer.

- **Rediscover Your Passions:** Reconnect with activities you enjoy, explore new interests, and set goals that bring you joy and purpose.

- **Focus on Gratitude:** Practice gratitude for the good things in your life, no matter how small. A grateful heart fosters a positive outlook and enhances your overall well-being.

- **Embrace Each Day:** Cancer can serve as a powerful reminder of the preciousness of life. Savor each day, cherish your relationships, and live life to the fullest.

The road ahead may not always be easy, but with hope, resilience, and a renewed appreciation for life, you can emerge from this experience stronger and more empowered than ever before.

This concludes Part 3 of this guide. Remember, you are not alone on this journey. There are many resources available to support you every step of the way. With knowledge, courage, and a positive outlook, you can face any challenge and thrive beyond cancer.

www.ingramcontent.com/pod-product-compliance
Lightning Source LLC
Chambersburg PA
CBHW050804250726
48653CB00006B/2063